CULINARY

CONCEPTIONS

NUTRIENT RICH RECIPES TO ENHANCE FEMALE FERTILITY

DR. ELIZABETH HYMANN

Copyright © 2023 by DR. ELIZABETH HYMANN

All rights reserved. No part of this publication may be reproduced, distributed, or transmitted in any form or by any means, including photocopying, recording, or other electronic or mechanical methods, without the prior written permission of the publisher, except in the case of brief quotations embodied in critical reviews and certain other noncommercial uses permitted by copyright law.

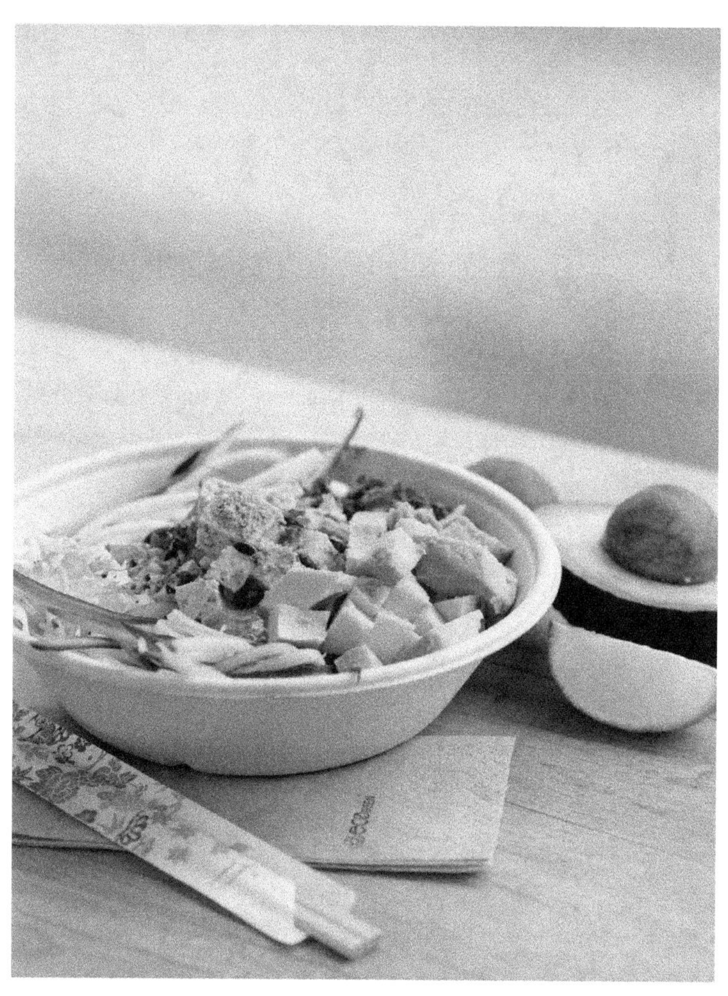

INTRODUCTION

In the pages of **"Culinary Conceptions: Nutrient-Rich Recipes to Enhance Female Fertility,"** a remarkable journey unfolds—a journey that transcends mere sustenance to embrace the profound intersection of nutrition and the delicate miracle of conception. This book is a guiding light for those who seek to nourish not only their bodies but also their aspirations, as they embark on a path towards enhanced female fertility.

Within these chapters, the symphony of flavors harmonizes with the science of well-being, offering a symposium of carefully crafted recipes that celebrate the art of nourishment. The introduction serves as the open door to this captivating narrative, inviting you to step into a world where food becomes a partner in the journey, where every bite carries the potential to shape the story of life itself.

As you embark on this culinary expedition, let the book be your compass, guiding you through the intricate tapestry of nutrients and their profound influence on reproductive health. It unveils the essence of key elements like folate, iron, omega-3 fatty acids, and antioxidants, each playing a vital role in creating an optimal environment for conception to flourish.

The book is more than words on a page; it's an invitation to transform your kitchen into a sanctuary of fertility, a canvas where nutrient-rich ingredients combine to create flavorful masterpieces. It weaves together the delicate threads of science and sensation, reminding you that every meal holds the potential to nourish not just your body, but your dreams as well.

As you turn the pages beyond the introduction, be prepared to embark on a sensory journey, where each recipe is a brushstroke in a painting of hope, and each dish a testament to the remarkable power of intention. "Culinary Conceptions" is not just a cookbook; it's a voyage of discovery, a celebration of life's most profound aspirations, and an ode to the transformative magic that happens when food becomes a partner in the dance of creation.

CHAPTER ONE

UNDERSTANDING FEMALE REPRODUCTIVE HEALTH

In the intricate mosaic of womanhood, the tapestry of female reproductive health is a masterpiece woven with threads of complexity, resilience, and profound beauty. As you venture into the heart of "Culinary Conceptions," a chapter dedicated to comprehending female reproductive health opens a portal into this captivating realm.

Within these pages, the book becomes a trusted guide, illuminating the inner workings of the female body's natural rhythms. Here, the symphony of hormones takes center stage, conducting an elegant dance that orchestrates fertility. With every turn of the page, you'll discover the ebb and flow of estrogen, the crescendo of luteinizing hormone, and the delicate embrace of progesterone – all harmonizing in a ballet that culminates in the potential for new life.

The introduction to female reproductive health is not merely a recitation of biological facts; it's an exploration of the exquisite artistry that defines a woman's journey. It unveils the enigma of the menstrual cycle, guiding you through its phases like chapters in a captivating novel. From the inception of menstruation to the threshold of ovulation, and from the secret preparations of the uterine lining to the poignant ballet of the corpus luteum – each stage is unveiled with a touch of reverence and awe.

But this exploration extends beyond the biological canvas; it acknowledges the emotional landscape that accompanies the journey. It recognizes the dreams that take flight like whispers on the wind, and the quiet strength required to navigate the currents of anticipation. This chapter stands as a gentle reassurance, reminding you that this voyage is not walked alone.

With each revelation, the understanding of your body deepens. The introduction casts a guiding light on fertility awareness, inviting you to decode the enigmatic signals that your body shares. It is an invitation to cultivate a partnership with your own physiology, to listen to the silent cues and embrace the rhythms that have been woven into your essence.

As you absorb the wisdom of this chapter, you become not just an observer, but an active participant in the symphony of life. This grants you the gift of knowledge, allowing you to attune yourself to the cadence of your fertility, to recognize the crescendos and decrescendos, and to step into the conductor's role of your own journey.

Female reproductive health encompasses a complex and intricate set of physiological processes that contribute to a woman's overall well-being and ability to conceive and bear children. Here's an overview of key aspects of female reproductive health:

1. Menstrual Cycle:

The menstrual cycle is a recurring monthly process that involves the release of an egg (ovulation), the preparation of the uterine lining for potential pregnancy, and the shedding of this lining if pregnancy does not occur (menstruation). The cycle is governed by hormonal fluctuations, primarily involving estrogen and progesterone.

2. Ovulation: Ovulation is the release of a mature egg from the ovary into the fallopian tube. This is a pivotal moment in the menstrual cycle, and it typically occurs around the middle of the cycle. Timing intercourse around ovulation is crucial for conception.

3. Hormones: Hormones play a central role in regulating the menstrual cycle and reproductive health. Estrogen and progesterone are key hormones that influence ovulation, fertility, and the maintenance of pregnancy.

4. Fertility Awareness: Fertility awareness methods involve tracking various bodily signs, such as basal body temperature, cervical mucus changes, and hormone levels, to determine the most fertile days of the

menstrual cycle. These methods can aid in contraception or conception planning.

5. Menstrual Health: Maintaining regular and healthy menstrual cycles is an indicator of reproductive health. Irregular cycles, heavy or painful periods, and other menstrual irregularities may signal underlying health issues.

6. Pregnancy: Female reproductive health also includes the ability to conceive, carry, and deliver a healthy pregnancy. Prenatal care, nutrition, and lifestyle choices are essential components of a healthy pregnancy.

7. Polycystic Ovary Syndrome (PCOS): PCOS is a hormonal disorder characterized by enlarged ovaries with small cysts. It can lead to irregular periods, fertility challenges, and other health concerns.

8. **Endometriosis**: Endometriosis occurs when tissue similar to the lining of the uterus grows outside the uterus. It can cause pain, heavy bleeding, and fertility problems.

9. **Pelvic Inflammatory Disease (PID)**: PID is an infection of the female reproductive organs, often caused by sexually transmitted infections. Left untreated, PID can lead to infertility.

10. **Fertility Challenges**: Infertility refers to the inability to conceive after a year of unprotected intercourse. Various factors can contribute to fertility challenges, including age, hormonal imbalances, and underlying health conditions.

11. **Perimenopause and Menopause**: As women age, their reproductive

system undergoes changes. Perimenopause refers to the transitional phase before menopause, which marks the end of a woman's reproductive years. Hormonal shifts during this time can lead to irregular periods and other symptoms.

12. Women's Health Screenings:

Regular gynecological check-ups and screenings, such as Pap smears and mammograms, are crucial for maintaining female reproductive health and detecting potential issues early.

As you proceed through the pages of this book, the understanding of female reproductive health becomes the compass that guides your choices, the cornerstone upon which you build your culinary journey. The recipes that follow, each a tribute to nourishment and intention, resonate with a deeper purpose as you honor the profound rhythms of womanhood and set forth on a path enriched with knowledge, empowerment, and the promise of life's exquisite potential.

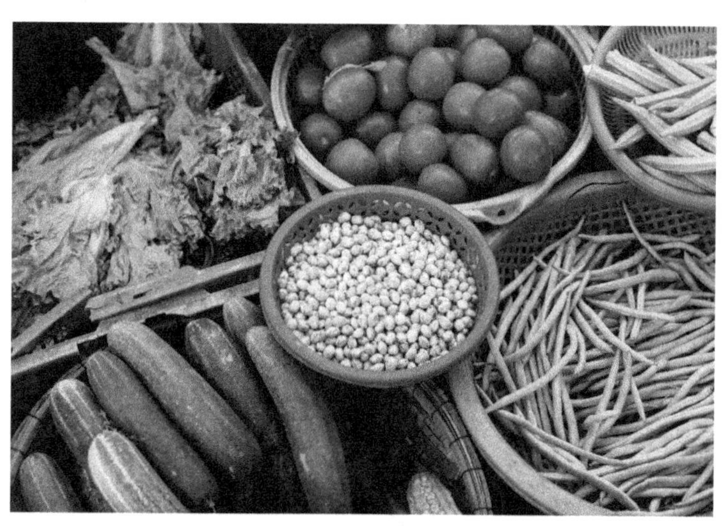

CHAPTER TWO

BUILDING A FOUNDATION: KEY NUTRIENTS FOR FERTILITY ENHANCEMENT

When embarking on a journey to enhance fertility, it's crucial to establish a solid nutritional foundation that supports the intricate processes of the female reproductive system. Key nutrients play a vital role in promoting hormonal balance, supporting cellular health, and facilitating the optimal conditions for conception. In this section, we delve into the essential nutrients that contribute to fertility enhancement.

Folate: Fueling Cell Division and Growth

Folate, a water-soluble B-vitamin, holds a pivotal role in promoting fertility and early embryonic development.

This nutrient aids in DNA synthesis and cell division, which are critical processes during the formation of a new life. Folate deficiency can lead to neural tube defects in the developing fetus, underscoring its importance before and during pregnancy. Leafy greens, citrus fruits, beans, and fortified grains are excellent dietary sources of folate.

Iron: Vitality and Oxygen Transport

Iron is a mineral with multifaceted importance in fertility. It supports healthy red blood cell production, ensuring optimal oxygen transport to tissues and organs, including the reproductive system. Iron deficiency, often resulting in anemia, can disrupt menstrual cycles and impair fertility. Incorporating iron-rich foods like lean meats, poultry, fish, beans, lentils, and dark leafy greens can help maintain healthy iron levels.

Omega-3 Fatty Acids: Inflammation Reduction and Hormonal Balance

Omega-3 fatty acids, particularly EPA (eicosapentaenoic acid) and DHA (docosahexaenoic acid), exhibit anti-inflammatory properties that contribute to reproductive health. They aid in regulating hormonal imbalances that can impact ovulation and overall fertility. These healthy fats can be sourced from fatty fish (such as salmon and mackerel), flaxseeds, chia seeds, and walnuts.

Vitamin D: Sunshine for Hormone Regulation

Vitamin D, often referred to as the "sunshine vitamin," plays a crucial role in fertility. It helps regulate hormones, supports immune function, and promotes healthy egg development. Inadequate vitamin D levels have been associated with irregular menstrual cycles and decreased fertility. Natural sources of vitamin D include sunlight exposure and dietary sources such as fatty fish, fortified dairy products, and egg yolks.

Antioxidants: Protecting Cellular Health

Antioxidants are powerful compounds that protect cells from oxidative stress, which can negatively impact fertility by damaging reproductive tissues. Vitamins C and E, selenium, and beta-carotene are examples of antioxidants that contribute to reproductive health. Including a variety of colorful fruits and vegetables, nuts, seeds, and whole grains in your diet provides a rich array of antioxidants.

By prioritizing these key nutrients, you're creating an environment within your body that nurtures reproductive health and enhances fertility. A well-balanced diet rich in folate, iron, omega-3 fatty acids, vitamin D, and antioxidants provides the building blocks necessary for optimal reproductive function. As you move forward on your fertility journey, remember that the foods you choose to nourish your body can have a profound impact on your overall well-being and the potential for conception.

Next, we'll explore how to set up your fertility-focused kitchen with essential ingredients that support your goal of enhancing fertility.

CHAPTER THREE

PREPARING YOUR FERTILITY KITCHEN: STOCKING ESSENTIALS

Let's delve into setting up your fertility-focused kitchen with essential ingredients.

Creating a fertility-enhancing culinary environment starts with a well-stocked kitchen that contains the essential ingredients to support your reproductive health goals. By having the right foods on hand, you'll be better equipped to prepare nutrient-rich meals that promote hormonal balance, cellular health, and overall fertility. In this section, we'll guide you through stocking your fertility kitchen with vital ingredients.

Whole Grains: The Foundation of Fertility

Whole grains are a cornerstone of a fertility-boosting diet. They provide a steady source of complex carbohydrates, which help regulate blood sugar levels and provide sustained energy. Opt for nutrient-dense grains like quinoa, brown rice, whole wheat pasta, and oats. These whole grains are rich in fiber, vitamins, and minerals that contribute to overall reproductive health.

Lean Proteins: Building Blocks for Fertility

Incorporating lean protein sources is essential for supporting hormone production and tissue repair. Choose lean options like poultry (skinless chicken or turkey), fish (salmon, cod, or sardines), lean cuts of beef or pork, and plant-based proteins such as beans, lentils, and tofu. These proteins provide amino acids that are crucial for cellular function and reproductive tissue development.

Healthy Fats: Hormonal Harmony

Healthy fats play a significant role in hormone production and regulation. Stock up on sources of monounsaturated and polyunsaturated fats like avocados, nuts (almonds, walnuts), seeds (flaxseeds, chia seeds), and olive oil. These fats support the absorption of fat-soluble vitamins and contribute to a healthy hormonal balance, aiding in ovulation and overall fertility.

Colorful Fruits and Vegetables: Antioxidant Powerhouses

Vibrant fruits and vegetables are packed with antioxidants and phytochemicals that protect reproductive cells from oxidative stress. Aim for a rainbow of colors to ensure a diverse intake of nutrients. Leafy greens (spinach, kale), berries, citrus fruits, carrots, sweet potatoes, and bell peppers are excellent choices to include in your fertility-focused kitchen.

Dairy or Dairy Alternatives: Calcium for Reproductive Health

Calcium is essential for reproductive health and bone density. Opt for dairy products like yogurt, kefir, and cheese, or choose fortified dairy alternatives like almond milk, soy milk, or coconut yogurt. These options provide calcium and vitamin D, both of which contribute to menstrual cycle regularity and overall reproductive function.

Herbs and Spices: Flavor and Functionality

Herbs and spices not only add flavor to your dishes but also offer potential health benefits. Cinnamon can help regulate blood sugar levels, while turmeric has anti-inflammatory properties. Ginger may aid digestion, and garlic can support immune function. Experiment with a variety of herbs and spices to enhance the nutritional value of your meals.

Nuts and Seeds: Snacking for Fertility

Nuts and seeds are nutrient-dense snacks that provide healthy fats, protein, and a variety of vitamins and minerals. Keep a variety of options on hand, such as almonds, walnuts, chia seeds, and sunflower seeds. These make for convenient and satisfying snacks that contribute to hormonal balance and reproductive health.

By stocking your fertility kitchen with these essential ingredients, you're setting the stage for nourishing meals that support your reproductive journey. Remember that a well-balanced and diverse diet, rich in whole foods and essential nutrients, plays a crucial role in enhancing fertility and promoting overall well-being.

In the upcoming sections, we'll explore nourishing breakfast, lunch, snack, dinner, and dessert options that incorporate these key ingredients to further boost your fertility-enhancing culinary repertoire.

CHAPTER FOUR

BREAKFAST BOOSTERS: MORNING MEALS FOR NOURISHING FERTILITY

Breakfast sets the tone for the day and plays a crucial role in supporting reproductive health. By starting your morning with nutrient-rich foods that promote hormonal balance and provide sustained energy, you're setting yourself up for a day of optimal well-being. In this section, we'll explore a variety of fertility-enhancing breakfast options that incorporate key ingredients to kickstart your day.

1. Berry Bliss Parfait: Antioxidant-Packed Start to Your Day

Indulge in the vibrant colors and flavors of a Berry Bliss Parfait. This breakfast option is brimming with antioxidants from berries, which protect reproductive cells from oxidative stress. Layer Greek yogurt or dairy-free yogurt with a mixture of mixed berries like blueberries, strawberries, and raspberries. Top with a sprinkle of granola for added crunch and a drizzle of honey for a touch of natural sweetness. Greek yogurt provides protein and calcium, while the berries contribute vitamins and minerals crucial for reproductive health.

Berry Bliss Parfait

Serves: One

Ingredients:

- Half cup of Greek yogurt
- One-quarter cup granola
- Half cup mixed berries (blueberries, strawberries, raspberries)
- One tablespoon honey or maple syrup
- One tablespoon chopped nuts (almonds, walnuts, or your choice)
- Fresh mint leaves for garnish (optional)

Instructions:

1. In a clear glass or jar, start by layering two tablespoons of Greek yogurt at the bottom.
2. Add a layer of one tablespoon of granola on top of the yogurt.
3. Add a layer of mixed berries (blueberries, strawberries, and raspberries).
4. Drizzle half teaspoon of honey or maple syrup over the berries.
5. Repeat the layers until you've used all the ingredients or reached the top of the glass.
6. Finish with a dollop of Greek yogurt on the top layer.

7. Sprinkle the chopped nuts on top for added crunch and nutrition.

8. Garnish with a fresh mint leaf if desired.

9. Serve immediately and enjoy your Berry Bliss Parfait!

This parfait is not only visually appealing but also packed with protein, fiber, antioxidants, and natural sweetness. Feel free to customize it with your favorite berries, nuts, and other additions like seeds or dried fruits.

2. Power Protein Pancakes: Fueling Hormone Production

Power Protein Pancakes

Serves: two-three (makes about six to eight pancakes)

Ingredients:

- One cup rolled oats (oat flour)

- One scoop (about 25 gram) protein powder (whey, plant-based, or your choice)

- One teaspoon baking powder

- Half teaspoon cinnamon (optional)

- One ripe banana

- Two large eggs

- One cup milk (dairy or non-dairy)

- One teaspoon vanilla extract

- Cooking spray or a bit of oil for cooking

Optional Add-ins:

- Chopped nuts (walnuts, almonds)

- Berries (blueberries, raspberries)

- Dark chocolate chips

Instructions:

1. In a blender or food processor, blend the rolled oats until they become a fine flour-like consistency.

2. Add the protein powder, baking powder, and cinnamon to the oat flour and pulse to combine.

3. In the same blender, add the ripe banana, eggs, milk, and vanilla extract. Blend until the mixture is smooth.

4. Combine the wet and dry ingredients in a bowl and stir until just combined. If you're adding optional ingredients like nuts, berries, or chocolate chips, fold them in gently.

5. Preheat a non-stick skillet or griddle over medium heat.

6. Lightly grease the skillet with cooking spray or a bit of oil.

7. Pour about half cup of batter onto the skillet for each pancake.

8. Cook until you see bubbles forming on the surface, then flip and cook for another one-two minutes, or until both sides are golden brown.

9. Repeat the process with the remaining batter.

10. Serve the Power Protein Pancakes warm with your choice of toppings, such as Greek yogurt, fresh berries, a drizzle of honey, or nut butter.

These protein-packed pancakes are not only delicious but also a great way to start your day with sustained energy. You can adjust the sweetness and flavor by adding more or less protein powder and experimenting with different toppings and mix-ins. Enjoy!

3. Green Goddess Smoothie: Nutrient-Rich Green Goodness

Energize your morning with a Green Goddess Smoothie that's brimming with fertility-boosting nutrients. Blend together a combination of leafy greens (spinach, kale), a variety of fruits (such as banana and pineapple), a source of healthy fat (like avocado), and a liquid base (such as almond milk). This nutrient-dense smoothie provides vitamins, minerals, antioxidants, and healthy fats that support hormonal balance and cellular health. Customize the ingredients to your taste preferences while ensuring a balanced nutritional profile.

Ingredients:

- One cup spinach (packed with nutrients)
- Half ripe banana (natural sweetness)

- Half avocado (healthy fats)
- Two cups pineapple chunks (vitamin C)
- Half cup cucumber (hydration)
- Half cup unsweetened almond milk (or your preferred milk)
- Half cup water (adjust for desired consistency)
- One tablespoon chia seeds (fiber, omega-3)
- Juice of half a lemon (bright flavor)
- Optional: a handful of ice cubes for extra chill

Instructions:

1. Add the spinach, banana, avocado, pineapple, cucumber, almond milk, and water to a blender.

2. Squeeze in the juice of half a lemon.

3. Add chia seeds for added fiber and omega-3 fatty acids.

4. If desired, add a handful of ice cubes to make the smoothie colder.

5. Blend on high until all the ingredients are smooth and well combined.

6. Taste and adjust the consistency or flavor by adding more water, lemon juice, or sweetener if needed.

7. Pour the Green Goddess Smoothie into a glass and enjoy immediately.

This smoothie is not only delicious but also incredibly nutrient-dense, providing a good balance of greens, healthy fats, vitamins, and hydration. Feel free to customize by adding other green vegetables, swapping fruits, or adjusting the liquid to suit your preferences.

4. Oatmeal with Seeds and Nuts:

Oats are a complex carbohydrate that can help regulate blood sugar levels, and seeds and nuts add healthy fats and nutrients.

Ingredients:

- one cup rolled oats

- one cup water or milk

- one tablespoon flaxseeds (source of omega-3s)

- one tablespoon pumpkin seeds (zinc)

- one tablespoon chopped walnuts (omega-3s)

- Half teaspoon cinnamon

- Sliced banana or other fruits for topping

Instructions:

1. Cook oats with water or milk until creamy.

2. Mix in flaxseeds, pumpkin seeds, chopped walnuts, and cinnamon.

3. Top with sliced banana or your favorite fruits.

5. Veggie Omelette:

Eggs are a source of high-quality protein and nutrients, while vegetables provide antioxidants and fiber.

Ingredients:

- Three eggs

- One-quarter cup diced bell peppers

- One-quarter cup diced spinach

- One-quarter cup diced tomatoes

- Salt and pepper to taste

- One teaspoon olive oil

Instructions:

1. Whisk eggs in a bowl with salt and pepper.

2. Heat olive oil in a skillet.

3. Add diced vegetables and sauté until tender.

4. Pour the whisked eggs into the skillet and cook until set.

5. Fold the omelette in half and serve.

6. Avocado Toast with Salmon:

Avocado provides healthy fats while salmon offers omega-3 fatty acids and protein, which can benefit fertility.

Ingredients:

- Two slices whole grain bread

- One ripe avocado

- Juice of half a lemon

- Salt and pepper to taste

- Smoked salmon slices

Instructions:

1. Mash avocado with lemon juice, salt, and pepper.

2. Toast the bread slices.

3. Spread the avocado mixture on the toast.

4. Top with smoked salmon slices.

7. Nut Butter and Banana Whole Grain Toast:

Whole grain bread offers complex carbs, while nut butter provides healthy fats and protein.

Ingredients:

- Two slices whole grain bread

- Two tablespoons nut butter (almond, peanut, etc.)

- One banana, sliced

- Honey drizzle (optional)

Instructions:

1. Toast the whole grain bread slices.

2. Spread nut butter on the toast.

3. Arrange sliced bananas on top.

4. Drizzle with honey if desired.

8. Quinoa Breakfast Bowl with Fruits:

Quinoa is a complete protein and contains important nutrients, and fruits provide vitamins and antioxidants.

Ingredients:

- Half cup cooked quinoa

- Half cup mixed berriesq (blueberries, strawberries, etc.)

- Half sliced kiwi

- One tablespoon chopped almonds

- One tablespoon unsweetened shredded coconut

- One teaspoon honey or agave syrup

Instructions:

1. Arrange cooked quinoa in a bowl.

2. Top with mixed berries, sliced kiwi, chopped almonds, and shredded coconut.

3. Drizzle with honey or agave syrup.

9. Spinach and Feta Breakfast Wrap:

Leafy greens like spinach provide folate, while eggs and feta cheese add protein and flavor.

Ingredients:

- Two large eggs

- One whole wheat tortilla

- Handful of baby spinach

- One-quarter cup crumbled feta cheese

- Salt and pepper to taste

- Salsa or hot sauce (optional)

Instructions:

1. Scramble eggs in a skillet with salt and pepper.

2. Warm the whole wheat tortilla.

3. Lay baby spinach on the tortilla.

4. Spoon scrambled eggs over the spinach.

5. Sprinkle crumbled feta cheese.

6. Roll up the tortilla and enjoy with salsa or hot sauce if desired.

10. Sweet Potato and Black Bean Breakfast Burrito:

Sweet potatoes offer beta-carotene, while black beans provide fiber and protein.

Ingredients:

- One small sweet potato, cooked and mashed

- Half cup black beans, drained and rinsed

- Two large eggs, scrambled

- One whole wheat tortilla

- Salsa or avocado slices for topping

- Salt and pepper to taste

Instructions:

1. Warm the whole wheat tortilla.

2. Spread mashed sweet potato on the tortilla.

3. Add scrambled eggs and black beans.

4. Season with salt and pepper.

5. Roll up the tortilla and serve with salsa or avocado slices.

Next up, we'll explore a variety of nourishing recipes for lunch, each carefully crafted to enhance fertility and provide the essential nutrients your body needs.

CHAPTER FIVE

LUNCHTIME LOVE: NUTRIENT-DENSE MIDDAY DELIGHTS

Lunch is an opportunity to refuel your body with essential nutrients that support reproductive health and overall well-being. Crafting nutrient-dense meals during this time not only sustains your energy levels but also provides your body with the necessary resources for optimal hormonal balance. In this section, we'll explore a selection of fertility-enhancing lunch options that incorporate key ingredients to nourish your body midday.

1. Quinoa and Avocado Salad: Plant-Based Protein Power

Elevate your lunch with a Quinoa and Avocado Salad that combines plant-based protein and healthy fats. Start with a base of cooked quinoa, which offers a complete protein source alongside essential amino acids. Add a variety of colorful vegetables such as cherry tomatoes, cucumbers, bell peppers, and red onion for a diverse range of vitamins and minerals. Top the salad with diced avocado for a dose of monounsaturated fats that support hormone production and absorption of fat-soluble vitamins.

Ingredients:

- One cup quinoa

- Two cups water or vegetable broth

- Two large ripe avocado, diced

- One cup cherry tomatoes, halved

- Half cucumber, diced

- One-quarter red onion, finely chopped

- One-quarter cup chopped fresh cilantro

- Juice of one lime

- Two tablespoons olive oil

- Salt and pepper to taste

Optional Add-ins:

- One-quarter cup crumbled feta cheese

- One-quarter cup chopped nuts (such as almonds or walnuts)

- One-quarter cup cooked black beans

Instructions:

1. Rinse the quinoa thoroughly under cold water.

2. In a saucepan, bring 2 cups of water or vegetable broth to a boil. Add the rinsed quinoa and a pinch of salt.

3. Reduce the heat to low, cover the saucepan, and let the quinoa simmer for about 15-20 minutes, or until the liquid is absorbed and the quinoa is cooked. Fluff the quinoa with a fork and let it cool.

4. In a large bowl, combine the cooked quinoa, diced avocado, halved cherry tomatoes, diced cucumber, finely chopped red onion, and chopped cilantro.

5. In a small bowl, whisk together the lime juice, olive oil, salt, and pepper to make the dressing.

6. Pour the dressing over the quinoa mixture and gently toss to combine all the ingredients.

7. If desired, add the optional add-ins like crumbled feta cheese, chopped nuts, or cooked black beans.

8. Taste and adjust the seasoning if needed.

9. Let the salad sit for about 10-15 minutes to allow the flavors to meld together.

10. Serve the Quinoa and Avocado Salad as a light and refreshing meal on its own or as a side dish.

This salad is a fantastic combination of protein-rich quinoa, healthy fats from avocado, and a burst of fresh flavors from the vegetables and herbs. Feel free to customize the salad by adding your favorite vegetables or proteins to make it even more satisfying.

2. Mediterranean Delight Wrap: Omega-3 Rich Mediterranean Flavors

Delight in the flavors of the Mediterranean with a nutrient-packed wrap. Fill a whole grain tortilla with a combination of ingredients like canned tuna or grilled chicken for lean protein. Add chopped olives, tomatoes, cucumbers, and feta cheese for a burst of flavor and nutrients. Drizzle with olive oil for healthy monounsaturated fats and a dose of omega-3 fatty acids. These fats support hormone regulation and reduce inflammation, contributing to reproductive health.

Ingredients:

- One whole wheat or spinach tortilla wrap

- One-quarter cup hummus (homemade or store-bought)

- One-quarter cup chopped cucumbers

- One-quarter cup chopped tomatoes

- One-quarter cup chopped red bell pepper

- One-quarter cup chopped red onion

- One-quarter cup crumbled feta cheese

- Two tablespoons chopped Kalamata olives

- Two tablespoons chopped fresh parsley

- One tablespoon extra-virgin olive oil

- Juice of half a lemon

- Salt and pepper to taste

- Optional: Grilled or canned salmon, flaked (for additional omega-3s)

Instructions:

1. In a small bowl, combine the chopped cucumbers, tomatoes, red bell pepper, and red onion.

2. Drizzle extra-virgin olive oil over the vegetables and squeeze the lemon juice over them.

3. Add a pinch of salt and pepper and toss to coat the vegetables in the dressing.

4. Lay the whole wheat or spinach tortilla wrap on a clean surface.

5. Spread a layer of hummus over the center of the wrap, leaving about an inch from the edges.

6. Spoon the prepared vegetable mixture over the hummus layer.

7. Sprinkle crumbled feta cheese and chopped Kalamata olives on top of the vegetables.

8. If using, add the grilled or canned salmon flakes.

9. Sprinkle chopped fresh parsley over the filling for a burst of flavor.

10. Fold in the sides of the tortilla and then roll it up tightly from the bottom, creating a wrap.

11. If desired, cut the wrap in half diagonally for easier handling.

12. Serve the Mediterranean Delight Wrap immediately as a satisfying and nutritious meal.

This wrap is a wonderful combination of Mediterranean flavors, providing healthy fats from olives and olive oil, omega-3s from salmon (if included), and a variety of colorful vegetables rich in vitamins and antioxidants. It's a perfect option for a quick and satisfying lunch or dinner.

3. Sweet Potato And Chickpea Buddha Bowl: Hormone-Happy Ingredients

Indulge in a Sweet Potato & Chickpea Buddha Bowl that's rich in nutrients known to support hormonal balance. Roasted sweet potatoes provide complex carbohydrates and beta-carotene, while chickpeas contribute plant-based protein and fiber. Add a generous portion of leafy greens like kale or spinach, and drizzle with tahini dressing for healthy fats and a touch of creaminess. The combination of ingredients ensures a well-rounded meal that promotes cellular health and overall fertility.

Ingredients:

- One large sweet potato, peeled and cubed

- One can (15 oz) chickpeas, drained and rinsed

- Two cups cooked quinoa or brown rice

- Two cups baby spinach or mixed greens

- Half avocado, sliced

- One-quarter cup pomegranate seeds (rich in antioxidants)

- One-quarter cup chopped walnuts (omega-3 fatty acids)

- Two tablespoons tahini (a source of healthy fats)

- Juice of one lemon

- One tablespoon olive oil

- One teaspoon ground turmeric (anti-inflammatory)

- Salt and pepper to taste

Instructions:

1. Preheat the oven to 400°F (200°C).

2. Toss the cubed sweet potato with olive oil, ground turmeric, salt, and pepper.

3. Spread the sweet potato cubes on a baking sheet and roast for about 20-25 minutes or until tender and slightly crispy.

4. In a small bowl, whisk together tahini, lemon juice, and a pinch of salt. Add a little water if needed to reach your desired consistency.

5. In a large bowl, assemble the Buddha bowl by layering cooked quinoa or brown rice, baby spinach or mixed greens, roasted sweet potato, chickpeas, sliced avocado, pomegranate seeds, and chopped walnuts.

6. Drizzle the tahini dressing over the top.

7. Sprinkle with additional salt, pepper, or lemon juice to taste.

8. Serve the Sweet Potato & Chickpea Buddha Bowl immediately as a satisfying and hormone-friendly meal.

This Buddha bowl is rich in a variety of nutrients that can promote hormonal balance and overall well-being. It's filled with fiber, healthy fats, antioxidants, and anti-inflammatory ingredients. Customize it by adding other hormone-supportive ingredients like flaxseeds, broccoli, and edamame, if desired.

4. Turkey and Avocado Lettuce Wraps: Lean Protein Kick

Lettuce wraps filled with lean turkey slices, creamy avocado, and a sprinkle of seeds for a protein-rich and refreshing lunch.

Ingredients:

- Large lettuce leaves (such as iceberg or butter lettuce)

- Sliced turkey breast

- Sliced avocado

- Sliced red bell peppers

- Chopped nuts (such as almonds or walnuts)

- Dijon mustard or your favorite dressing for drizzling

Instructions:

1. Lay lettuce leaves on a clean surface.

2. Place sliced turkey breast, sliced avocado, and sliced red bell peppers on each leaf.

3. Sprinkle chopped nuts over the filling.

4. Drizzle with Dijon mustard or your favorite dressing.

5. Fold the sides of the lettuce leaf to create a wrap.

5. Spinach and Chickpea Salad with Balsamic Vinaigrette: Green Power

A nutrient-packed salad combining leafy greens, protein-rich chickpeas, and a flavorful balsamic vinaigrette.

Ingredients:

- Two cups baby spinach

- One cup cooked chickpeas

- One-quarter cup cherry tomatoes, halved

- One-quarter cup diced cucumber

- One-quarter red onion, thinly sliced

- Two tablespoons crumbled feta cheese

- Balsamic vinaigrette: Two tablespoons balsamic vinegar, one tablespoon olive oil, one teaspoon Dijon mustard, salt, and pepper to taste

Instructions:

1. In a large bowl, combine baby spinach, chickpeas, cherry tomatoes, diced cucumber, and red onion.

2. In a separate bowl, whisk together balsamic vinegar, olive oil, Dijon mustard, salt, and pepper to make the dressing.

3. Drizzle the dressing over the salad and toss to combine.

4. Top with crumbled feta cheese and enjoy.

6. Grilled Salmon Salad: Omega-3 Rich

Elevate your lunchtime with the delightful and nourishing Grilled Salmon Salad. Packed with the goodness of omega-3 fatty acids, this salad combines the succulent flavors of grilled salmon with an array of vibrant vegetables and a zesty Lemon-Dijon Dressing. The marriage of omega-3 rich salmon, nutrient-rich greens, and a burst of tangy dressing creates a harmonious and satisfying dish that's not only a treat for your taste buds but also a nutritional boost for your overall well-being.

Ingredients:

- Two salmon fillets (6-8 oz each)

- Four cups mixed greens (such as baby spinach, arugula, and lettuce)

- One cup cherry tomatoes, halved

- Half cucumber, sliced

- One-quarter red onion, thinly sliced

- One-quarter cup feta cheese, crumbled

- One-quarter cup chopped walnuts or almonds (for added omega-3s)

- Olive oil for grilling

- Salt and pepper to taste

For the Lemon-Dijon Dressing:

- Three tablespoons olive oil

- Two tablespoons lemon juice

- One teaspoon Dijon mustard

- One teaspoon honey or maple syrup (optional)

- Salt and pepper to taste

Instructions:

1. Preheat the grill to medium-high heat.

2. Brush the salmon fillets with a little olive oil and season with salt and pepper.

3. Grill the salmon fillets for about 4-5 minutes per side, or until cooked through and flaky. Cooking time may vary based on the thickness of the fillets.

4. While the salmon is grilling, prepare the Lemon-Dijon Dressing by whisking together olive oil, lemon juice, Dijon mustard, honey or maple syrup (if using), salt, and pepper in a small bowl.

5. In a large bowl, combine mixed greens, cherry tomatoes, sliced cucumber, and red onion.

6. Toss the salad with a portion of the Lemon-Dijon Dressing. Adjust the amount according to your taste.

7. Divide the dressed salad onto serving plates.

8. Once the grilled salmon fillets are ready, place one fillet on each salad plate.

9. Sprinkle crumbled feta cheese and chopped walnuts or almonds over the salads.

10. Drizzle a little more dressing over the salmon and the rest of the salad.

11. Serve the Grilled Salmon Salad immediately as a delicious and omega-3 rich meal.

This salad not only provides a healthy dose of omega-3 fatty acids from the salmon and nuts but also incorporates a variety of fresh vegetables for a well-rounded and flavorful meal. Feel free to customize the ingredients or dressing to suit your preferences.

7. Tofu and Veggie Stir-Fry

A protein-packed stir-fry with tofu, an excellent source of plant-based protein, and an array of colorful vegetables.

Ingredients:

- One cup cubed tofu

- Assorted stir-fry vegetables (broccoli, snap peas, bell peppers, etc.)

- Two tablespoons soy sauce or tamari

- One teaspoon sesame oil

- One clove garlic, minced

- One teaspoon ginger, minced

- Cooked brown rice or quinoa for serving

Instructions:

1. Heat sesame oil in a skillet or wok over medium heat.

2. Add minced garlic and ginger and sauté for a minute.

3. Add tofu and stir-fry until lightly browned.

4. Add the vegetables and cook until tender-crisp.

5. Pour in soy sauce or tamari and stir to coat.

6. Serve the stir-fry over cooked brown rice or quinoa.

8. Lentil and Vegetable Stew

A comforting stew loaded with protein-packed lentils and a mix of colorful vegetables for a hearty and wholesome lunch.

Ingredients:

- One cup cooked green or brown lentils

- Assorted diced vegetables (carrots, celery, zucchini, etc.)

- Vegetable broth

- One clove garlic, minced

- One teaspoon ground cumin

- Half teaspoon turmeric

- Salt and pepper to taste

- Chopped fresh parsley for garnish

Instructions:

1. In a pot, sauté minced garlic, ground cumin, and turmeric until fragrant.

2. Add diced vegetables and cook for a few minutes.

3. Pour in vegetable broth and cooked lentils.

4. Simmer until vegetables are tender.

5. Season with salt and pepper.

6. Garnish with chopped fresh parsley and serve.

9. Whole Grain Pasta Salad with Pesto and Veggies

A refreshing pasta salad tossed with homemade pesto, assorted veggies, and whole grain pasta for a light yet satisfying option.

Ingredients:

- One cup cooked whole grain pasta

- Assorted chopped veggies (cherry tomatoes, bell peppers, olives, etc.)

- Pesto sauce (store-bought or homemade)

- Chopped fresh basil for garnish

- Lemon zest for added flavor

Instructions:

1. In a bowl, combine cooked whole grain pasta and chopped veggies.

2. Toss with pesto sauce until well coated.

3. Garnish with chopped fresh basil and lemon zest.

4. Serve at room temperature or chilled.

10. Chickpea Stir-Fry

Chickpea Stir-Fry offers a burst of plant-powered goodness that combines the rich creaminess of chickpeas with an array of vibrant stir-fry vegetables. This dish effortlessly marries together the hearty protein of chickpeas and a medley of colorful vegetables, creating a harmonious symphony of textures and flavors. Tossed in a savory sesame-infused sauce, this stir-fry offers a delightful balance between nutrition and taste.

Ingredients:

- One can (15 oz) chickpeas, drained and rinsed

- Two cups mixed stir-fry vegetables (bell peppers, snap peas, broccoli, carrots, etc.)

- Two tablespoons soy sauce or tamari (use gluten-free if needed)

- One teaspoon sesame oil

- One clove garlic, minced

- One teaspoon minced ginger

- Cooked brown rice or quinoa for serving

Optional Add-ins:

- Sliced scallions

- Crushed red pepper flakes for heat

- Sesame seeds for garnish

Instructions:

1. Heat the sesame oil in a large skillet or wok over medium-high heat.

2. Add minced garlic and minced ginger to the skillet and sauté for about 1 minute until fragrant.

3. Add the mixed stir-fry vegetables tto the skillet. Stir-fry for 3-4 minutes until they start to become tender but still crisp.

4. Add the drained and rinsed chickpeas to the skillet and continue to stir-fry for an additional 2-3 minutes to heat them through.

5. Pour in the soy sauce or tamari over the chickpeas and vegetables. Toss everything together to coat well.

6. If using, add sliced scallions and crushed red pepper flakes for extra flavor and heat.

7. Once everything is heated and coated in the sauce, remove the skillet from the heat.

8. Serve the chickpea stir-fry over cooked brown rice or quinoa.

9. Garnish with sesame seeds if desired.

Enjoy this Chickpea Stir-Fry for a quick, flavorful, and plant-based meal rich in protein, fiber, and essential nutrients. You can customize the vegetables and seasoning to suit your taste preferences.

These lunchtime options demonstrate the potential of midday meals to contribute to your reproductive health journey by incorporating nutrient-dense ingredients. By selecting ingredients that support hormonal balance, provide essential nutrients, and offer sustained energy, you're making a positive impact on your overall well-being.

In the upcoming section, we'll explore nourishing recipes for energizing snacks, satisfying dinners, and delightful desserts, each carefully curated to enhance fertility and provide the building blocks your body needs.

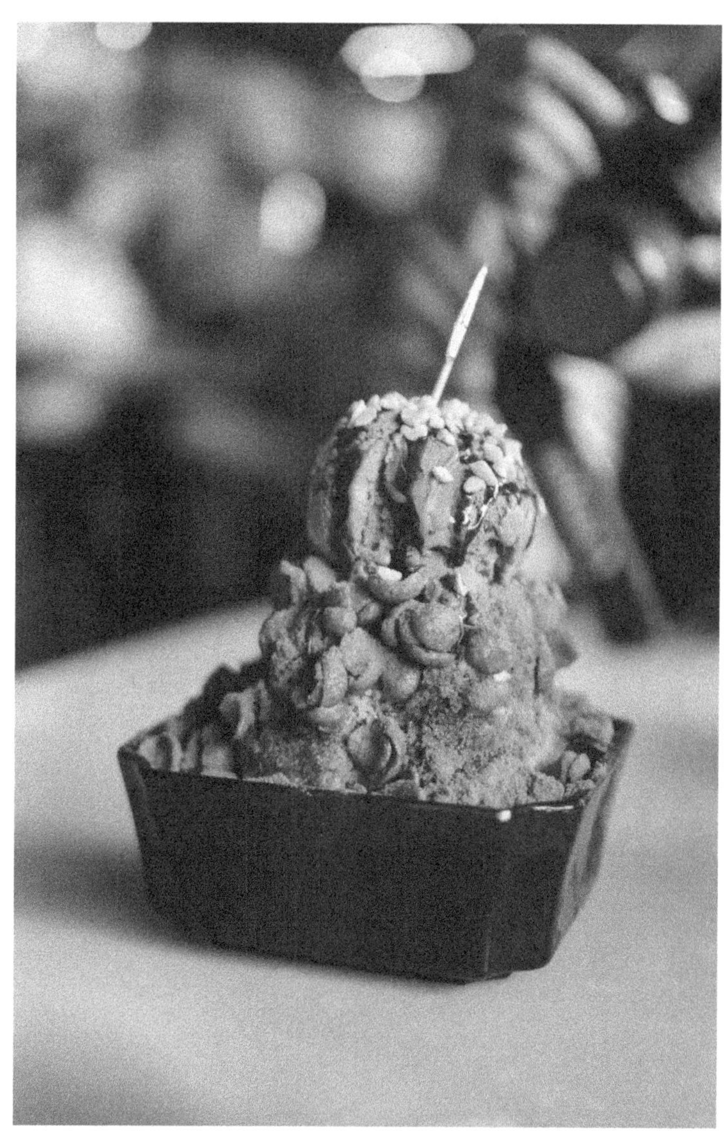

CHAPTER SIX

ENERGIZING SNACKS: SUSTAINING YOUR FERTILITY THROUGHOUT THE DAY

Between meals, it's important to refuel your body with nutrient-rich snacks that provide sustained energy and support your reproductive health goals. Smart snacking can help regulate blood sugar levels, maintain hormonal balance, and prevent energy crashes. In this section, we'll explore a variety of fertility-enhancing snack options that incorporate key ingredients to keep you energized throughout the day.

Nutty Energy Bites: Nourishing On-the-Go Treats

Prepare Nutty Energy Bites in advance for a convenient and nourishing snack option. Combine ingredients like rolled oats, nut butter (such as almond or peanut butter), honey, chia seeds, and a touch of dark chocolate chips for a hint of sweetness. These bites provide a combination of healthy fats, protein, and fiber, which contribute to sustained energy and hormonal balance. Pack them for on-the-go nourishment or enjoy them as a midday pick-me-up.

Hummus & Veggie Dippers: Fiber-Packed Snacking

Create a satisfying snack by pairing homemade or store-bought hummus with an array of colorful veggie dippers. Carrot sticks, cucumber slices, bell pepper strips, and cherry tomatoes make for excellent companions to creamy hummus. Hummus offers plant-based protein, while the vegetables provide vitamins, minerals, and dietary fiber that supports digestive health and hormone regulation.

Roasted Almond Trail Mix: Portable Nutrient Powerhouse

Craft a customized Roasted Almond Trail Mix by combining almonds, walnuts, dried fruits (like cranberries or apricots), and a sprinkle of seeds (such as pumpkin or sunflower seeds). This nutrient-dense mix offers a balance of healthy fats, protein, and antioxidants, making it a versatile snack option. The mix is not only satisfying but also contributes to reproductive health by providing essential nutrients and energy.

Other Healthy Snack Choices Include:

1. Berries with Greek Yogurt: Enjoy a bowl of Greek yogurt topped with a mix of antioxidant-rich berries like blueberries, strawberries, and raspberries.

2. Hard-Boiled Eggs: Hard-boiled eggs are a great source of protein and healthy fats, making them a convenient and nutritious snack.

3. Apple Slices with Nut Butter: Pair apple slices with almond or peanut butter for a delicious blend of fiber, natural sweetness, and healthy fats.

4. Chia Seed Pudding: Prepare chia seed pudding using almond milk and top it with fresh fruit for a nutrient-rich snack loaded with omega-3s and fiber.

5. Avocado Toast: Top whole grain toast with mashed avocado and a sprinkle of seeds for a combination of healthy fats, fiber, and vitamins.

6. Cottage Cheese with Pineapple: Enjoy cottage cheese with a side of pineapple for a protein-rich and vitamin C-packed snack.

7. Trail Mix: Create a custom trail mix with a mix of nuts, seeds, dried fruits, and dark chocolate chips for a balance of flavors and nutrients.

8. Yogurt Parfait: Layer yogurt with granola, chopped fruits, and a drizzle of honey for a satisfying and probiotic-rich snack.

9. Dark Chocolate and Almonds: A small serving of dark chocolate paired with almonds offers a dose of antioxidants and healthy fats.

10. Roasted Chickpeas: Season and roast chickpeas in the oven for a crunchy and protein-packed snack.

11. Smoothie: Blend a smoothie with spinach, frozen berries, banana, Greek yogurt, and a splash of almond milk for a nutrient-packed refreshment.

14. Seaweed Snacks: Enjoy crispy seaweed snacks for a low-calorie option rich in minerals and antioxidants.

15. *Edamame:* Steamed or roasted edamame pods provide plant-based protein and essential nutrients.

In the upcoming section, we'll continue to explore recipes for nourishing dinners, each carefully designed to provide the nutrients your body needs on your fertility journey.

CHAPTER SEVEN

NOURISHING DINNERS: SATISFYING SUPPERS FOR FERTILITY ENHANCEMENT

Dinner is an opportunity to wind down and nourish your body with a satisfying meal that supports reproductive health and overall well-being. Crafting nutrient-dense dinners not only satiates your hunger but also ensures that your body receives the essential nutrients it needs for optimal hormonal balance.

In this section, we'll explore a variety of fertility-enhancing dinner options that incorporate key ingredients to nourish you at the end of the day.

1. Salmon and Asparagus Delight: Omega-3 Feast

Indulge in the richness of omega-3 fatty acids with a Salmon and Asparagus Delight. This dinner option features a baked or grilled salmon fillet, which is rich in EPA and DHA, essential fatty acids that support hormonal balance and reduce inflammation. Serve the salmon alongside roasted asparagus, a source of antioxidants and fiber. Add a side of quinoa or brown rice for complex carbohydrates and a complete protein profile.

Ingredients:

- Two salmon fillets (6-8 oz each)
- One bunch asparagus, trimmed
- Two tablespoons olive oil
- Two cloves garlic, minced
- Lemon zest and juice from 1 lemon

- Salt and pepper to taste

- Fresh dill or parsley for garnish

Instructions:

1. Preheat the oven to 400°F (200°C).

2. Place the salmon fillets on a baking sheet lined with parchment paper.

3. In a small bowl, mix together olive oil, minced garlic, lemon zest, lemon juice, salt, and pepper.

4. Brush the olive oil mixture over the salmon fillets, coating them evenly.

5. Arrange the trimmed asparagus around the salmon on the baking sheet.

6. Drizzle a little olive oil over the asparagus and season with salt and pepper.

7. Bake in the preheated oven for about 12-15 minutes, or until the salmon is cooked through and flakes easily with a fork.

8. While baking, you can baste the salmon with any remaining olive oil mixture for extra flavor.

9. Once cooked, remove from the oven and garnish with fresh dill or parsley.

10. Serve the Salmon and Asparagus Delight alongside your favorite side dish, such as quinoa, brown rice, or a mixed salad.

This recipe offers a delicious and nutritious combination of omega-3 rich salmon and fiber-packed asparagus, along with the bright flavors of lemon and herbs. Adjust the cooking time based on the thickness of the salmon fillets. Enjoy this simple yet satisfying dinner that's perfect for a balanced and fertility-supporting meal.

2. Spinach and Lentil Curry: Plant-Based Hormone Support

Embrace plant-based protein and aromatic flavors with a Spinach and Lentil Curry. Lentils are a fantastic source of protein, fiber, and essential nutrients that support hormone production and cellular health. Combine them with spinach, tomatoes, and a blend of curry spices for a satisfying and nutrient-packed meal. Serve your curry with whole grain naan or brown rice for a well-rounded dinner that enhances reproductive wellness.

Ingredients:

- One cup green or brown lentils, rinsed and drained
- One onion, finely chopped
- Two cloves garlic, minced
- One-inch piece of ginger, grated
- One teaspoon cumin seeds
- One teaspoon ground turmeric
- One teaspoon ground coriander
- Half teaspoon ground cumin
- Half teaspoon chili powder (adjust to taste)
- Half teaspoon garam masala
- One-quarter teaspoon ground cinnamon
- One-quarter teaspoon ground cardamom
- One can (14 oz) diced tomatoes

- One can (14 oz) coconut milk

- Four cups fresh spinach leaves, washed and chopped

- Two tablespoons olive oil

- Salt and pepper to taste

- Fresh cilantro for garnish

- Cooked rice or naan bread for serving

Instructions:

1. In a large pot, heat the olive oil over medium heat. Add the cumin seeds and let them sizzle for a minute until fragrant.

2. Add the chopped onion and sauté until it becomes translucent.

3. Stir in the minced garlic and grated ginger, cooking for about a minute until fragrant.

4. Add the ground turmeric, ground coriander, ground cumin, chili powder, garam masala, ground cinnamon, and ground cardamom. Stir the spices into the onion mixture to form a fragrant paste.

5. Pour in the diced tomatoes and coconut milk. Stir well to combine the ingredients.

6. Add the rinsed lentils to the pot and stir to coat them with the tomato and coconut mixture.

7. Pour in enough water to cover the lentils and bring the mixture to a boil. Once boiling, reduce the heat to low, cover the pot, and let it simmer for about 20-25 minutes, or until the lentils are tender.

8. Stir in the chopped spinach and let it wilt into the curry.

9. Season the curry with salt and pepper to taste. Adjust the chili powder if you prefer more or less heat.

10. Once the lentils are cooked and the spinach is wilted, remove the pot from the heat.

11. Serve the Spinach and Lentil Curry over cooked rice or with naan bread.

12. Garnish with fresh cilantro for added flavor and freshness.

This Spinach and Lentil Curry is a flavorful and nutrient-rich dish that combines the earthy flavors of lentils and aromatic spices with the vibrant freshness of spinach. Enjoy this comforting and wholesome meal as part of a fertility-supporting dinner.

3. Grilled Chicken Quinoa Bowl: Balanced Nutrient Boost

Create a balanced dinner with a Grilled Chicken Quinoa Bowl that offers a medley of flavors and nutrients. Grill or bake a chicken breast marinated in herbs and spices for lean protein. Prepare quinoa as the base, and top it with a variety of roasted or sautéed vegetables such as bell peppers, zucchini, and carrots. Drizzle with a vinaigrette made from olive oil and lemon juice for healthy fats that support hormone regulation.

Ingredients:

For the Grilled Chicken:

- Two boneless, skinless chicken breasts
- Two tablespoons olive oil
- One teaspoon dried oregano
- One teaspoon garlic powder
- Salt and pepper to taste

For the Quinoa Bowl:

- One cup quinoa

- Two cups water or chicken broth

- Two cups mixed greens or baby spinach

- One cup cherry tomatoes, halved

- One cucumber, diced

- One red bell pepper, diced

- One-quarter red onion, thinly sliced

- Kalamata olives (optional)

- Feta cheese (optional)

For the Lemon-Dijon Dressing:

- One-quarter cup olive oil

- Two tablespoons lemon juice

- One teaspoon Dijon mustard

- One teaspoon honey or maple syrup

- Salt and pepper to taste

Instructions:

For the Grilled Chicken:

1. Preheat the grill to medium-high heat.

2. In a bowl, mix olive oil, dried oregano, garlic powder, salt, and pepper to create a marinade.

3. Coat the chicken breasts with the marinade on both sides.

4. Grill the chicken for about 6-7 minutes per side, or until cooked through and the internal temperature reaches 165°F (74°C). Cooking time may vary based on the thickness of the chicken breasts.

5. Once cooked, remove the chicken from the grill and let it rest for a few minutes before slicing.

For the Quinoa Bowl:

1. Rinse the quinoa under cold water.

2. In a saucepan, bring the water or chicken broth to a boil. Add the rinsed quinoa, reduce the heat to low, cover, and simmer for about 15 minutes, or until the quinoa is cooked and the liquid is absorbed.

3. Fluff the cooked quinoa with a fork and let it cool slightly.

For the Lemon-Dijon Dressing:

1. In a small bowl, whisk together olive oil, lemon juice, Dijon mustard, honey or maple syrup, salt, and pepper until well combined.

Assembling the Grilled Chicken Quinoa Bowl:

1. In individual serving bowls, layer mixed greens or baby spinach as the base.

2. Top the greens with cooked quinoa, cherry tomatoes, diced cucumber, diced red bell pepper, and thinly sliced red onion.

3. Arrange the sliced grilled chicken on top of the quinoa and vegetables.

4. If using, add Kalamata olives and crumbled feta cheese.

5. Drizzle the Lemon-Dijon Dressing over the bowl.

6. Serve the Grilled Chicken Quinoa Bowl immediately, and enjoy the balanced flavors and textures.

This Grilled Chicken Quinoa Bowl offers a blend of lean protein, whole grains, and vibrant vegetables, all tied together with a zesty dressing. Feel free to customize the ingredients and dressing according to your taste preferences and dietary needs.

4. Whole Wheat Pasta Primavera

Ingredients:

- Two cups cooked whole wheat pasta
- One cup mixed vegetables (e.g., cherry tomatoes, broccoli, bell peppers)
- One tablespoon olive oil
- Two cloves garlic, minced
- One-quarter cup grated Parmesan cheese
- One tablespoon chopped fresh parsley
- Lemon zest
- Salt and pepper to taste

Instructions:

- Sauté mixed vegetables in olive oil until tender.

- Add minced garlic and sauté for another minute.

- Toss cooked pasta with sautéed vegetables.

- Mix in grated Parmesan cheese, chopped parsley, and lemon zest.

- Season with salt and pepper before serving.

5. Blackberry Walnut Salad with Grilled Turkey

Ingredients:

- Two grilled turkey cutlets, sliced

- Four cups mixed greens

- One cup blackberries

- Half cup crumbled blue cheese

- One-quarter cup chopped walnuts

- Balsamic vinaigrette dressing

Instructions:

- Toss mixed greens, blackberries, blue cheese, and walnuts in a bowl.

- Top with sliced grilled turkey.

- Drizzle with balsamic vinaigrette before serving.

6. Berry-Almond Chia Pudding

Ingredients:

- One-quarter cup chia seeds

- One cup almond milk (or any milk of your choice)

- Half teaspoon vanilla extract

-Mixed berries (e.g., strawberries, blueberries, raspberries)

- Sliced almonds for topping

Instructions:

- Mix chia seeds, almond milk, and vanilla extract in a jar.

- Stir well and refrigerate overnight or for at least 2 hours, until it thickens.

- Layer chia pudding with mixed berries and sliced almonds before serving.

7. Sweet Potato and Black Bean Tacos

Ingredients:

- Two medium sweet potatoes, peeled and cubed

- One can black beans, drained and rinsed

- One teaspoon cumin

- One teaspoon chili powder

- Half teaspoon paprika

- Whole wheat tortillas

- Avocado slices, salsa, and plain Greek yogurt for toppings

Instructions:

- Roast sweet potato cubes with spices until tender.

- Warm black beans and season with a bit of cumin and chili powder.

- Fill tortillas with sweet potatoes, black beans, and desired toppings.

8. Salmon and Asparagus Foil Packets

Ingredients:

- Two salmon fillets

- One bunch asparagus, trimmed

- One lemon, thinly sliced

- Fresh dill sprigs

- Salt and pepper to taste

- Olive oil

Instructions:

- Place salmon fillets on sheets of aluminum foil.

- Arrange asparagus and lemon slices around the salmon.

- Drizzle with olive oil; season with salt, pepper, and dill.

- Seal foil packets and bake at 400°F (200°C) for 15-20 minutes.

9. Roasted Beet and Goat Cheese Salad

Ingredients:

- Two medium beets, roasted, peeled, and sliced

- Four cups mixed greens

- One-quarter cup crumbled goat cheese

- One-quarter cup chopped walnuts or pistachios

- Balsamic vinaigrette dressing

Instructions:

- Arrange mixed greens on plates.

- Top with roasted beet slices, crumbled goat cheese, and chopped nuts.

- Drizzle with balsamic vinaigrette before serving.

10. Broccoli and Mushroom Quiche with Whole Wheat Crust

Ingredients:

Ingredients for the Crust:

- One and Half cups whole wheat flour

- One-quarter teaspoon salt

- Half cup cold unsalted butter, diced

- Four to five tablespoons ice water

Ingredients for the Filling:

- Two cups broccoli florets, blanched and chopped

- One cup sliced mushrooms

- Half cup shredded cheddar cheese

- Four large eggs

- One cup milk (dairy or non-dairy)

- Salt, pepper, and nutmeg to taste

Instructions:

- In a food processor, pulse flour and salt.

- Add diced butter and pulse until mixture resembles coarse crumbs.

- Gradually add ice water and pulse until dough comes together.

- Roll out dough and fit into a pie pan; refrigerate for Thirty minutes.

- Preheat oven to 375°F (190°C).

- Arrange blanched broccoli and sliced mushrooms on the crust.

- Sprinkle shredded cheese over the vegetables.

- In a bowl, whisk eggs, milk, salt, pepper, and a pinch of nutmeg.

- Pour egg mixture over the vegetables and cheese.

- Bake for Thirty-five to Forty minutes or until the quiche is set and golden.

11. Spaghetti Squash with Turkey Bolognese

Ingredients:

- One medium spaghetti squash

- One pound ground turkey

- One can crushed tomatoes

- One onion, chopped

- Two cloves garlic, minced

- One teaspoon dried oregano

- One teaspoon dried basil

- Salt and pepper to taste

- Grated Parmesan cheese for topping

Instructions:

- Preheat oven to 375°F (190°C).

- Cut spaghetti squash in half lengthwise and scoop out seeds.

- Place squash halves face-down on a baking sheet; bake for 30-40 minutes, until tender.

- In a skillet, cook ground turkey until browned; drain excess fat.
- Add chopped onion and minced garlic; cook until onion is translucent.
- Stir in crushed tomatoes, oregano, basil, salt, and pepper.
- Simmer sauce for about 15-20 minutes.
- Use a fork to scrape the spaghetti squash into "noodles."
- Serve the turkey Bolognese sauce over the spaghetti squash noodles and top with grated Parmesan cheese.

These dinner options showcase the potential of evening meals to contribute to your reproductive health journey through the incorporation of nutrient-dense ingredients. By selecting ingredients that support hormonal balance, provide essential nutrients, and offer satisfying flavors, you're making a positive impact on your overall well-being.

In the upcoming sections, we'll continue to explore recipes for sweet indulgences, fertility-boosting beverages, and lifestyle tips that complement your fertility-enhancing dietary choices.

CHAPTER EIGHT

SWEET INDULGENCIES: DESSERTS WITH A FERTILITY FOCUS

Satisfying your sweet tooth while supporting your reproductive health goals is entirely possible with the right dessert choices. Desserts can be crafted to incorporate nutrient-rich ingredients that contribute to hormonal balance, provide essential vitamins and minerals, and offer a guilt-free indulgence. In this section, we'll explore a variety of fertility-enhancing dessert options that use key ingredients to create delightful treats.

1. Almond Butter and Banana Energy Bites

Ingredients:

- One cup rolled oats

- Half cup almond butter

- One-quarter cup honey or maple syrup

- One ripe banana, mashed

- Half teaspoon vanilla extract

- Pinch of salt

- Unsweetened shredded coconut or chopped nuts for coating (optional)

Instructions:

1. In a bowl, mix rolled oats, almond butter, honey or maple syrup, mashed banana, vanilla extract, and a pinch of salt.

2. Roll the mixture into small balls.

3. Optional: Roll the energy bites in unsweetened shredded coconut or chopped nuts to coat.

4. Place the energy bites on a plate or tray and refrigerate for about 30 minutes to firm up.

5. Enjoy these energy bites as a satisfying and nutrient-rich dessert.

2. Baked Apples with Cinnamon and Walnuts

Ingredients:

- Two apples, cored and halved

- Two tablespoons chopped walnuts

- One teaspoon cinnamon

- One teaspoon honey or maple syrup

- Greek yogurt or cottage cheese for serving (optional)

Instructions:

1. Preheat the oven to 350°F (175°C).

2. Place the apple halves on a baking sheet, cut side up.

3. In a bowl, mix chopped walnuts, cinnamon, and honey or maple syrup.

4. Fill the apple halves with the walnut mixture.

5. Bake for about Twenty to Twenty-five minutes, or until the apples are tender.

6. Serve the baked apples warm, optionally topped with a dollop of Greek yogurt or cottage cheese.

3. Mixed Berry Frozen Yogurt

Ingredients:

- Two cups mixed berries (e.g., strawberries, blueberries, raspberries)
- Two cups plain Greek yogurt
- One-quarter cup honey or agave syrup
- One teaspoon vanilla extract

Instructions:

1. Blend the mixed berries until smooth.

2. In a bowl, combine the berry puree, Greek yogurt, honey or agave syrup, and vanilla extract.

3. Pour the mixture into an ice cream maker and churn according to the manufacturer's instructions.

4. Transfer the frozen yogurt to a container and freeze for an additional hour to firm up.

5. Scoop and enjoy this refreshing and creamy frozen yogurt.

4. Mango and Coconut Chia Popsicles

Ingredients:

- One ripe mango, peeled and pitted

- One can coconut milk (full-fat)

- Two tablespoons chia seeds

- One tablespoon honey or agave syrup (optional)

Instructions:

1. Blend the mango until smooth.

2. In a bowl, combine the blended mango, coconut milk, chia seeds, and sweetener if desired.

3. Pour the mixture into popsicle molds.

4. Freeze for at least 4 hours or until solid.

5. Enjoy these tropical chia popsicles as a refreshing dessert.

5.   Dark   Chocolate-Dipped Strawberries

Ingredients:

- Fresh strawberries, washed and dried

- Dark chocolate (70% cocoa or higher)

- Chopped nuts (e.g., almonds, pistachios) or shredded coconut (optional)

Instructions:

1. Melt the dark chocolate in a microwave or over a double boiler.

2. Hold each strawberry by the stem and dip it into the melted chocolate, coating about half of the strawberry.

3. Optional: Roll the dipped part of the strawberry in chopped nuts or shredded coconut for added texture and flavor.

4. Place the dipped strawberries on a parchment-lined tray and let them cool until the chocolate hardens.

5. Enjoy these indulgent chocolate-dipped strawberries in moderation.

6. *Banana and Walnut Oat Cookies*

Ingredients:

- Two ripe bananas, mashed

- One and half cups old-fashioned oats

- One-quarter cup chopped walnuts

- One-quarter cup dried cranberries or raisins

- One teaspoon cinnamon

- Half teaspoon vanilla extract

Instructions:

1. Preheat the oven to 350°F (175°C) and line a baking sheet with parchment paper.

2. In a bowl, mix mashed bananas, oats, chopped walnuts, dried cranberries or raisins, cinnamon, and vanilla extract.

3. Scoop spoonfuls of the mixture onto the baking sheet, shaping them into cookies.

4. Bake for about Fifteen to Twenty minutes, or until the cookies are golden and firm.

5. Allow the cookies to cool before enjoying these naturally sweet treats.

7. Pumpkin Spice Chia Pudding

Ingredients:

- 1/4 cup chia seeds

- 1 cup almond milk (or any milk of your choice)

- 1/4 cup pumpkin puree

- 1 tablespoon maple syrup or honey

- 1/2 teaspoon pumpkin spice blend

- Chopped pecans or pumpkin seeds for topping

Instructions:

1. Mix chia seeds, almond milk, pumpkin puree, maple syrup or honey, and pumpkin spice in a bowl.

2. Stir well and refrigerate for at least 2 hours or until the mixture thickens.

3. Top with chopped pecans or pumpkin seeds before serving.

8. Chocolate Avocado Mousse

Ingredients:

- Two ripe avocados, peeled and pitted

- One-quarter up cocoa powder (unsweetened)

- One-quarter cup honey or maple syrup

- One teaspoon vanilla extract

- Pinch of salt

- Fresh berries for topping

Instructions:

1. Blend avocados, cocoa powder, honey or maple syrup, vanilla extract, and a pinch of salt until smooth.

2. Spoon the mousse into serving bowls or glasses.

3. Chill in the refrigerator for at least 30 minutes.

4. Top with fresh berries before serving.

9. Coconut Date Energy Balls

Ingredients:

- One cup pitted dates

- Half cup shredded coconut (unsweetened)

- Half cup rolled oats

- One-quarter cup almond butter

- One-quarter cup chopped almonds or cashews

- One teaspoon vanilla extract

- Pinch of salt

Instructions:

1. Blend dates, shredded coconut, rolled oats, almond butter, chopped nuts, vanilla extract, and a pinch of salt in a food processor until the mixture forms a sticky dough.

2. Roll the mixture into small balls.

3. Refrigerate for about 30 minutes to firm up.

4. Enjoy these naturally sweet energy balls as a satisfying dessert.

Remember, enjoying these desserts in moderation as part of a balanced diet can be a delightful way to incorporate fertility-supportive ingredients. If you have specific dietary requirements or concerns, consider consulting with a healthcare professional or registered dietitian.

CHAPTER NINE

Fertility-Boosting Beverages: Hydration with a Purpose

Hydration is an essential pillar of reproductive health, and the beverages you choose can play a significant role in enhancing fertility. By carefully selecting ingredients that support hormonal balance, provide essential nutrients, and offer antioxidants, you can nourish your body and create an environment conducive to conception. In this section, we'll explore a variety of fertility-boosting beverages designed to provide hydration with a purpose.

Herbal Infusions for Hormonal Harmony

Embrace the power of nature's botanicals with Herbal Infusions that offer hormonal support. Herbs like red clover, raspberry leaf, nettle, and chasteberry (vitex) are renowned for their potential to regulate menstrual cycles, promote reproductive wellness, and nurture hormonal harmony. Prepare these infusions by steeping a combination of dried herbs in hot water for an extended period, allowing their beneficial compounds to infuse the liquid. Sip on these infusions as warm or cold beverages to provide your body with gentle herbal assistance on your fertility journey.

Green Tea Elixir: Supporting Reproductive Wellness

Discover the antioxidant-rich goodness of a Green Tea Elixir, a beverage celebrated for its potential to support reproductive health. Brew green tea leaves in hot water and infuse the elixir with a squeeze of lemon juice to bolster the absorption of tea's antioxidants. The catechins in green tea offer cellular protection and may positively influence ovulation. As you savor this elixir, you're nurturing your body with compounds that contribute to hormonal balance and overall reproductive well-being.

Fertility Smoothie Creations: Customizable Nutrient Blends

Embark on a flavorful journey with Fertility Smoothie Creations, where you have the power to tailor nutrient-rich ingredients into a delicious beverage. Start with a liquid base, whether it's almond milk, coconut water, or a dairy-free option. Incorporate leafy greens, such as spinach or kale, for a vitamin and mineral boost. Add a medley of fruits like berries, banana, and mango to infuse natural sweetness and antioxidants. Elevate your smoothie with fertility-friendly additions like chia seeds, flaxseeds, and a scoop of high-quality protein powder. With a whirl of the blender, you create a customizable elixir that not only tantalizes your taste buds but also nourishes your body in line with your reproductive health goals.

The beverages you choose to consume on your fertility journey can contribute to the holistic approach you've taken to enhance reproductive wellness. By thoughtfully selecting ingredients that support hormonal balance and overall health, you're actively nurturing your body's readiness for conception.

CHAPTER TEN

BEYOND THE PLATE: LIFESTYLE TIPS FOR FERTILITY ENHANCEMENT

Enhancing fertility isn't solely about dietary choices; it involves adopting a holistic approach that encompasses various aspects of your lifestyle. From stress management to exercise and prioritizing restful sleep, every facet of your daily routine can influence your reproductive health journey. In this section, we'll explore lifestyle tips that go beyond the plate, offering insights into fostering a well-rounded and fertile environment within your body.

Stress Management: Finding Balance for Reproductive Health

Chronic stress can disrupt hormonal balance and negatively impact fertility. Prioritize stress management techniques such as meditation, deep breathing, yoga, and mindfulness. Engaging in these practices helps lower cortisol levels, regulate hormones, and create a more fertile environment. Finding moments of tranquility and practicing stress reduction can play a significant role in supporting your reproductive well-being.

Exercise and Fertility: Movement for Hormonal Harmony

Regular physical activity is crucial for maintaining a healthy weight and promoting hormonal balance. Engage in moderate exercise, such as walking, swimming, or cycling, to support blood flow to reproductive organs and encourage regular ovulation. However, avoid excessive exercise that might lead to irregular menstrual cycles. Striking the right balance between movement and rest contributes to optimal reproductive function.

Sleep and Relaxation: Prioritizing Rest for Conception

Quality sleep is essential for overall health and fertility. Create a sleep-friendly environment, establish a regular sleep schedule, and aim for 7-9 hours of restorative sleep each night. Proper sleep helps regulate hormone production, supports immune function, and contributes to the body's natural rhythm. Prioritizing sleep and incorporating relaxation techniques can positively impact your fertility journey.

Mindfulness and Emotional Well-Being: Nurturing a Positive Mindset

Cultivating a positive mindset and emotional well-being can create a harmonious environment for conception. Practice mindfulness, engage in activities you enjoy, and foster connections with loved ones. Stress and anxiety can influence hormone levels, so maintaining emotional equilibrium is paramount. Building emotional resilience and nurturing your mental health contributes to your holistic approach to fertility enhancement.

Environmental Toxins: Minimizing Exposure for Reproductive Health

Limit exposure to environmental toxins that can disrupt hormonal balance. Choose organic produce when possible to reduce exposure to pesticides, and opt for non-toxic household and personal care products. Avoid excessive alcohol and tobacco consumption, as these substances can impact fertility. Being mindful of environmental factors and making conscious choices contributes to creating a fertile environment.

Medical Consultation: Partnering with Healthcare Professionals

While lifestyle changes play a significant role in fertility enhancement, it's crucial to partner with healthcare professionals. Consult with a healthcare provider, such as a gynecologist or reproductive endocrinologist, to address any underlying medical conditions or concerns. A comprehensive approach that combines lifestyle adjustments and medical guidance can optimize your chances of successful conception.

By integrating these lifestyle tips into your daily routine, you're creating a supportive and nurturing environment for your fertility journey. A holistic approach that encompasses stress management, exercise, sleep, emotional well-being, environmental considerations, and medical support paves the way for enhanced reproductive health.

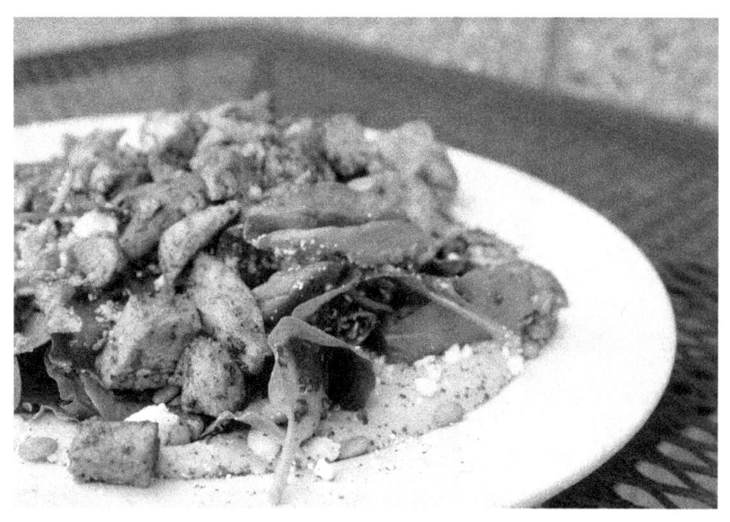

CONCLUSION

Congratulations on completing your culinary journey to enhanced female fertility!

Throughout this guide, you've gained valuable insights into the intersection of nutrition and reproductive health. By incorporating nutrient-rich ingredients into your meals and making mindful lifestyle choices, you've taken proactive steps towards optimizing your reproductive well-being. As you reflect on your journey, let's recap the key takeaways and celebrate the empowering knowledge you've acquired.

Nourishing Your Reproductive Health

You've learned that nutrition plays a pivotal role in supporting reproductive health. By focusing on whole grains, lean proteins, healthy fats, colorful fruits, and vegetables, you've nourished your body with essential nutrients that promote hormonal balance, cellular health, and overall fertility. These foods not only provide sustenance but also create a favorable environment for conception and reproductive wellness.

Delightful and Nutrient-Packed Meals

From breakfast to dinner and even indulgent desserts, you've discovered a plethora of recipes that incorporate fertility-enhancing ingredients. Whether it's the omega-3 fatty acids in salmon, the antioxidants in berries, or the fiber in legumes, each meal was crafted with care to contribute to your reproductive health goals. These meals exemplify the harmonious blend of taste and nutrition that is the cornerstone of your fertility-focused culinary journey.

Hydration with Intention

Your choice of beverages is not just about quenching thirst; it's an opportunity to provide your body with additional nourishment. Whether sipping on herbal infusions for hormonal balance, enjoying a green tea elixir for its antioxidants, or blending nutrient-packed smoothies, you've embraced hydration as a means to enhance your fertility journey from within.

Lifestyle as a Holistic Approach

Beyond the plate, you've recognized that a holistic approach to fertility encompasses more than just dietary choices. Stress management, regular exercise, quality sleep, emotional well-being, and minimizing exposure to environmental toxins all contribute to creating a fertile environment. By nurturing your body and mind, you've taken comprehensive steps towards fostering reproductive health and overall well-being.

Partnering with Professionals

You've understood the importance of partnering with healthcare professionals to ensure a well-rounded approach to fertility enhancement. Consulting with medical experts allows you to address any underlying medical conditions, receive personalized guidance, and ensure that your holistic efforts are aligned with your individual needs.

As you conclude this culinary journey, remember that each meal you prepare, each ingredient you select, and each lifestyle choice you make contributes to your reproductive health journey. Your knowledge, choices, and efforts have the power to impact your well-being in profound ways.

Remember that your journey is unique, and every step you take brings you closer to your goals. Embrace this journey with positivity, patience, and the knowledge that you're empowering yourself on the path to enhanced female fertility.

www.ingramcontent.com/pod-product-compliance
Lightning Source LLC
Chambersburg PA
CBHW070852260726
48661CB00004B/1358